My Beautiful Teeth Series

Part 3

A Visit to the Dentist

Dr. Tasneem Mahmoud Omran

- My Beautiful Teeth Series
- Part 3: A Visit to the Dentist
- Dr. Tasneem Mahmoud Omran
- First Edition
- All rights are reserved to the author

About this Series: Discovering the World of Dental Health

My Beautiful Teeth Series is a comprehensive and engaging guide to dental health for children aged 5-7. This 3-part series is designed to educate and inspire children to take care of their teeth, while also raising awareness about the importance of oral hygiene.

1- Tiny but Mighty: Explores the importance of teeth and how they help us talk and eat properly. It also teaches children about the different types of teeth and why babies don't have any teeth when they are born.

2- Let's Take Care of Our Teeth: Focuses on the proper techniques for brushing and flossing, as well as the importance of eating healthy foods for strong teeth.

3- A Visit to the Dentist: Takes children on a journey to the dental clinic, where they learn about the different tools and equipment used by dentists and the importance of regular check-ups.

Each book in the series contains interactive games and activities, including connect-the-dots and matching exercises that will keep children engaged and entertained while learning about dental health. Additionally, a QR code included in each book, allows children to play each game in an interactive way using their mobile phone or tablet.

"My Beautiful Teeth Series" is a must-have for any parent looking to educate their children about dental health in a fun and engaging way.

Meet the Dentist: Our Teeth's Best Friend

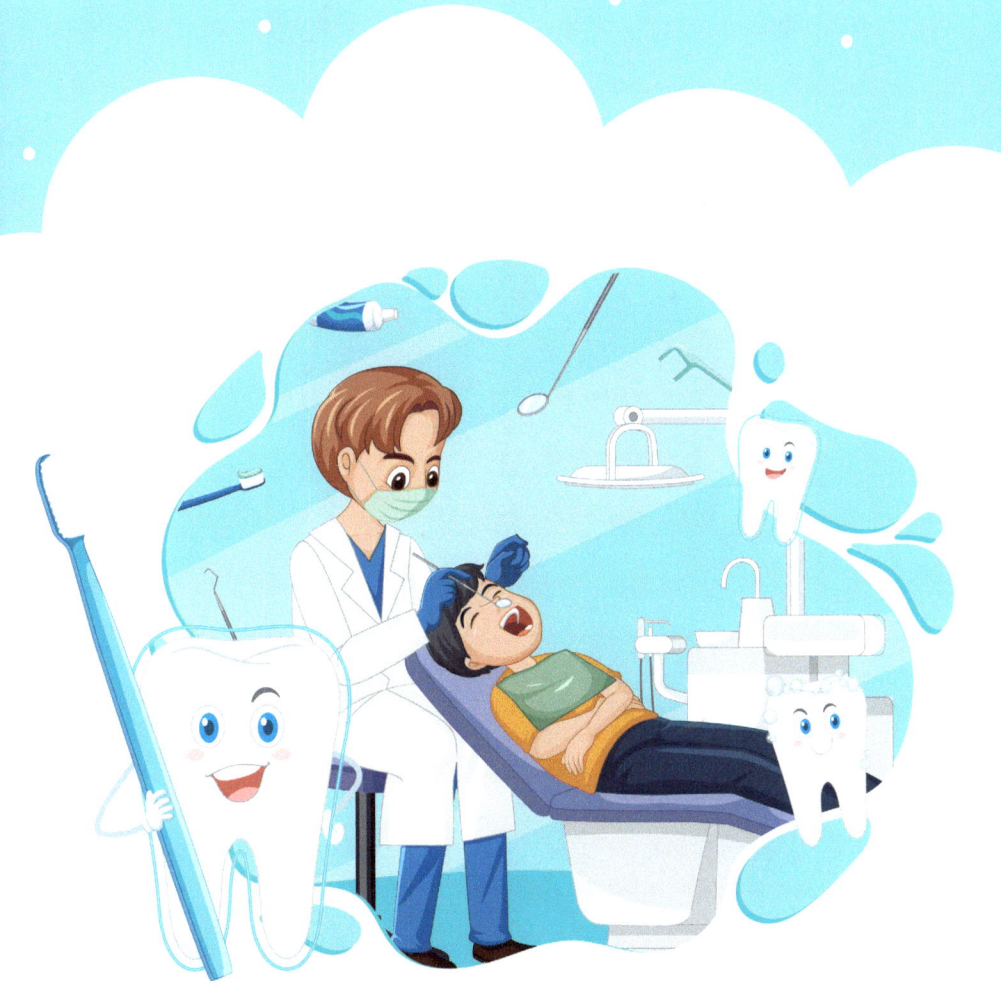

Why it is important to visit the dentist?

The Dentist is a special doctor who takes care of our teeth and mouths.

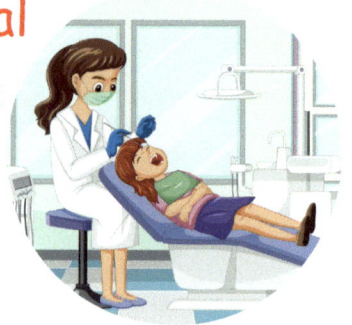

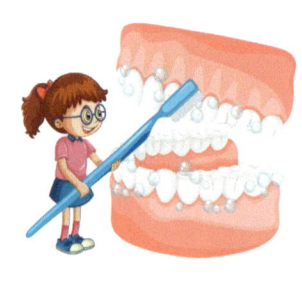

They help us keep our teeth strong. They also teach us the right ways to brush and take care of them.

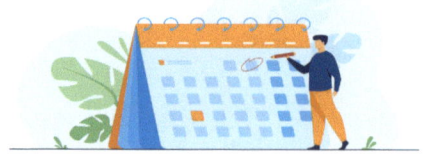

We should visit the dentist regularly, about twice a year.

What does the Dentist do?

The Dentist checks your teeth and makes sure you're brushing them properly.

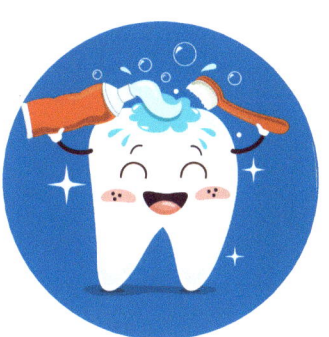

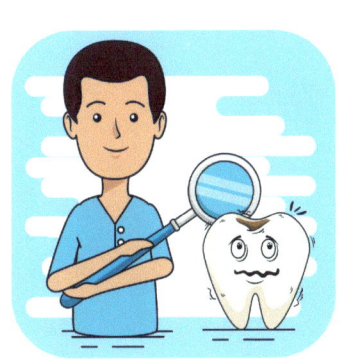

They also check to see if your teeth are growing in the right way, and look for cavities.

If you have cavities, the dentist will take care of them.

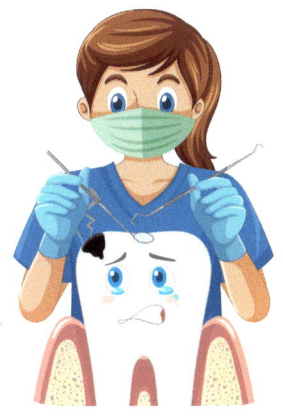

Your dentist also checks your tongue and the inside of your mouth to make sure everything is healthy.

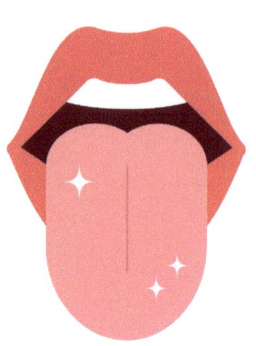

If you have any questions about your teeth or how to take care of them, ask your dentist.

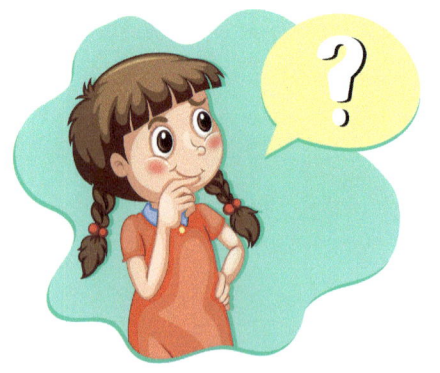

Your dentist is a friendly doctor who wants you to have healthy, shiny teeth.

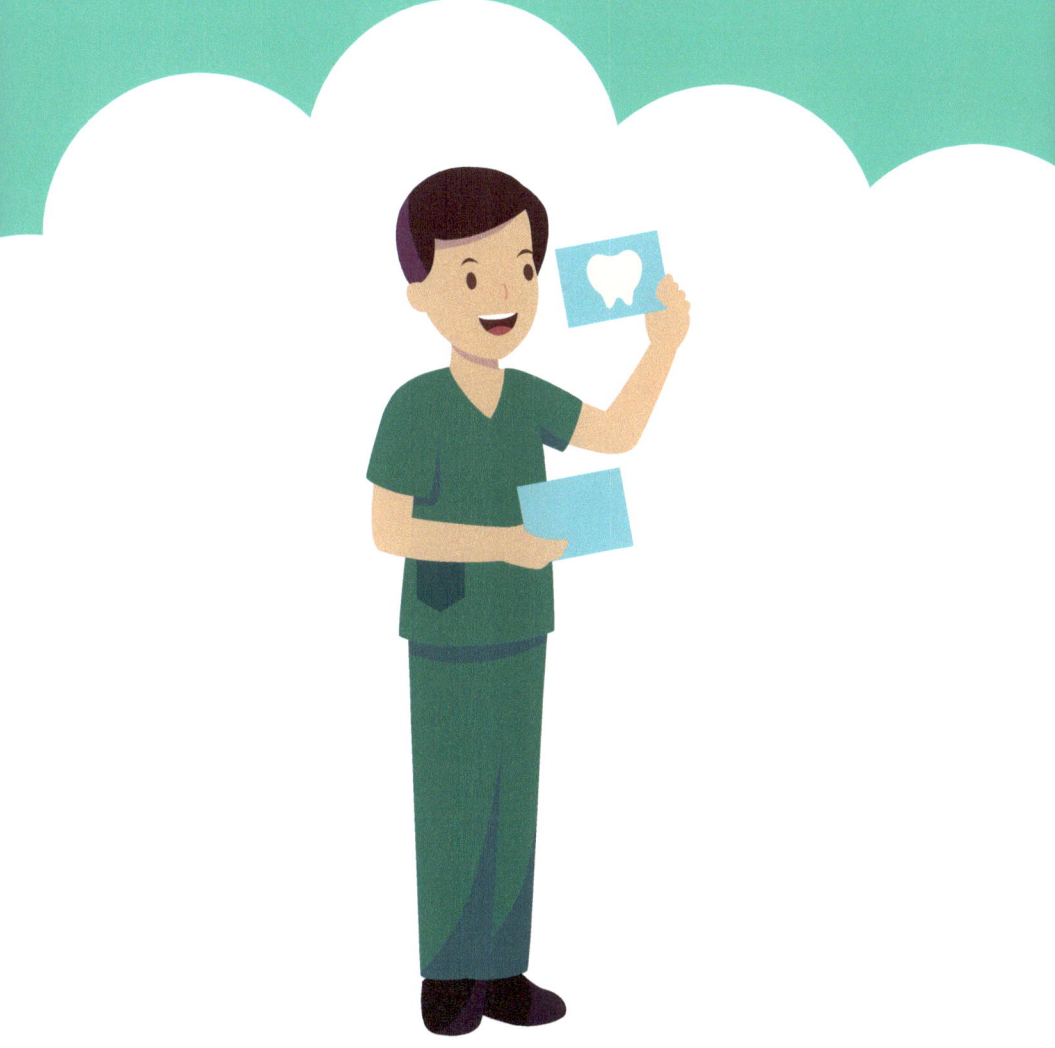

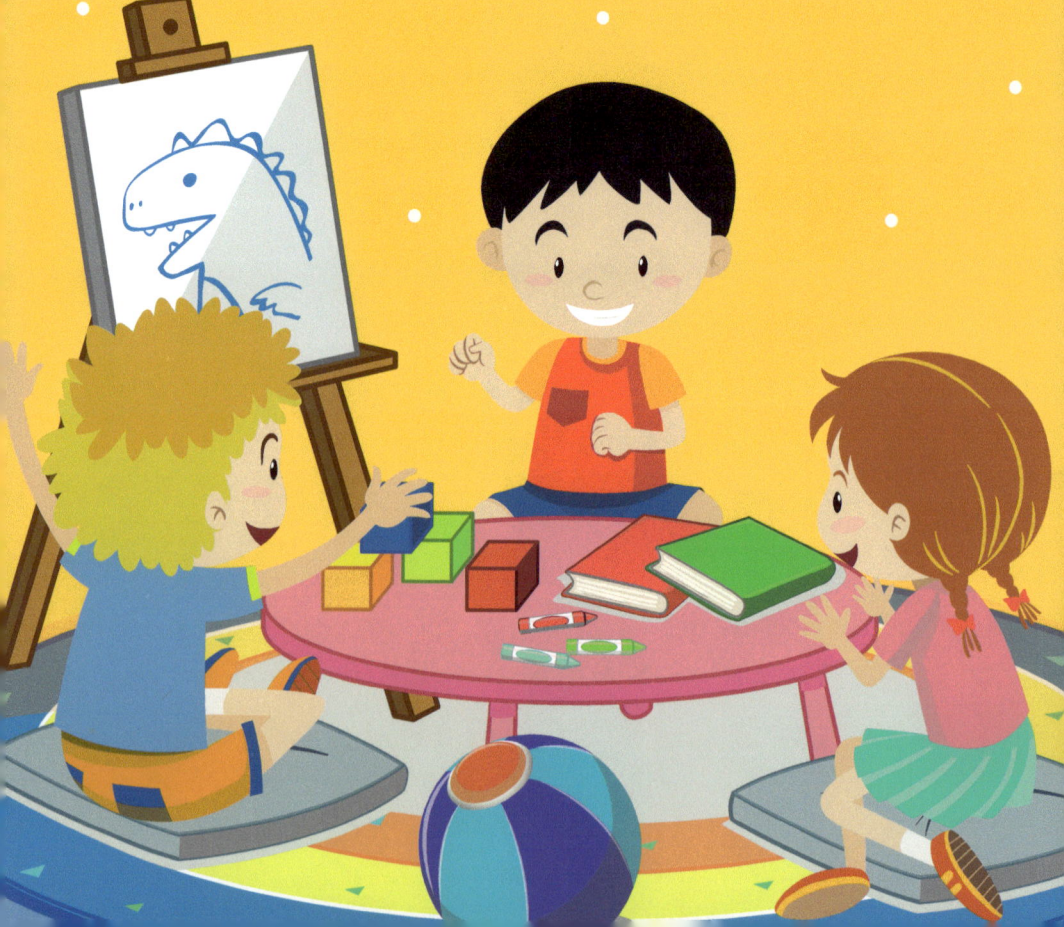

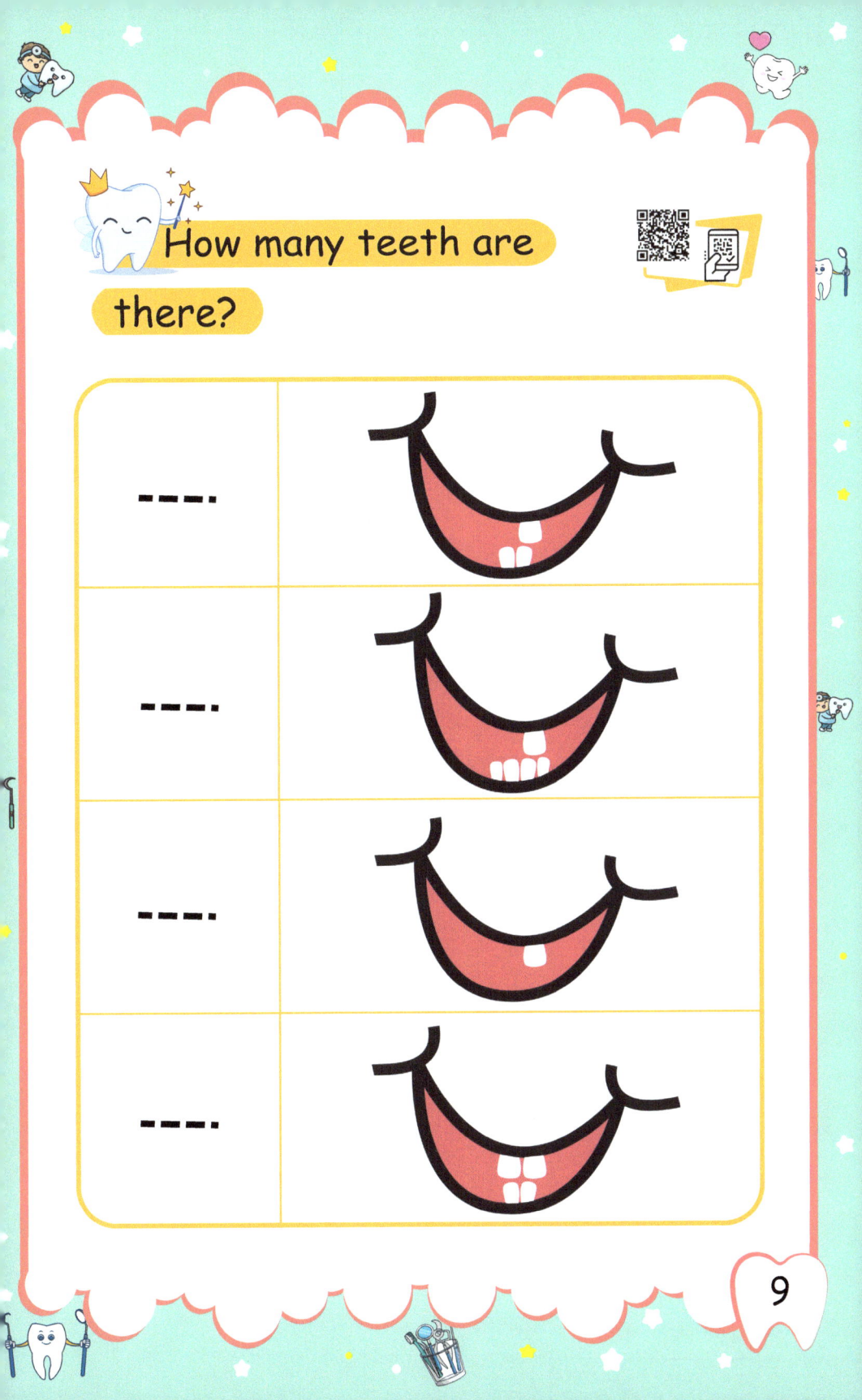

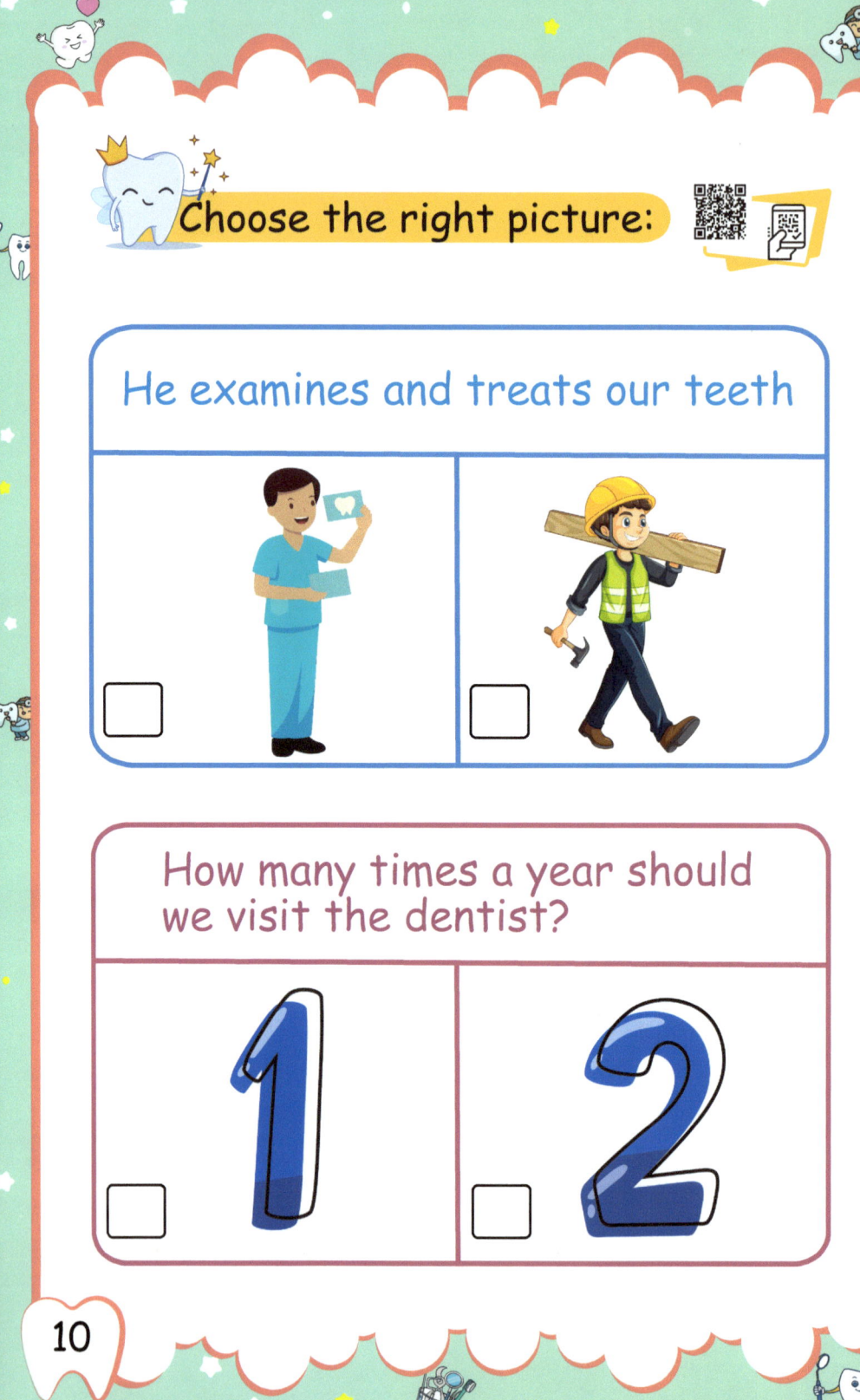

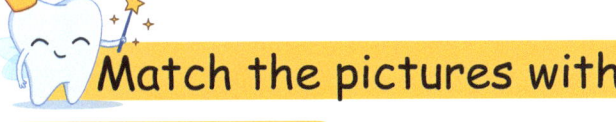 Match the pictures with their shadows:

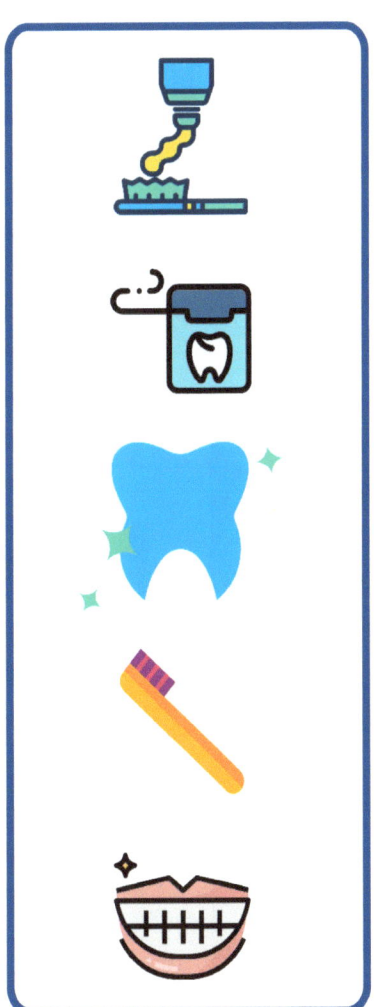

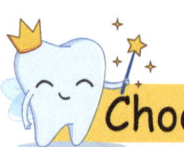
Choose the two missing pieces to complete the picture:

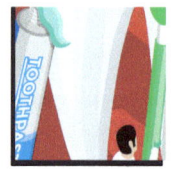
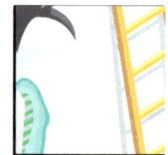
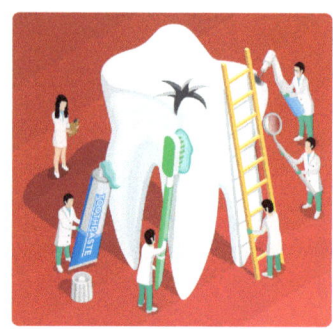

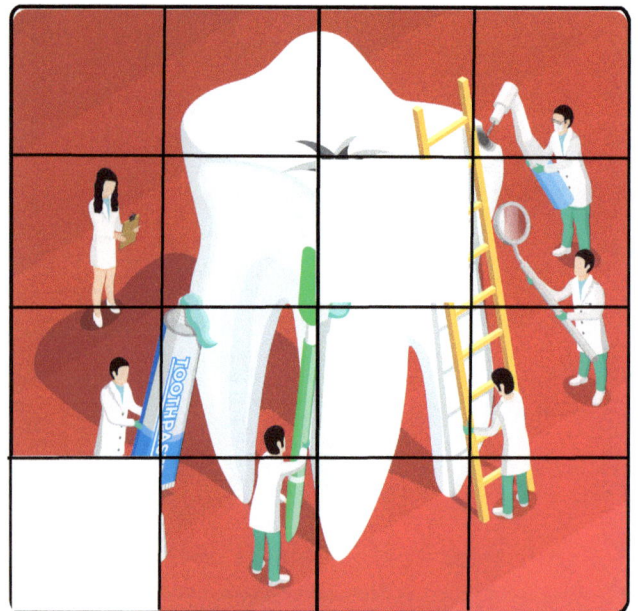

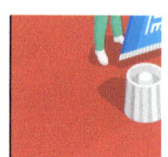

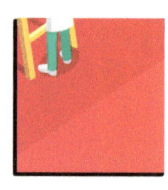

Exploring the Dental Clinic

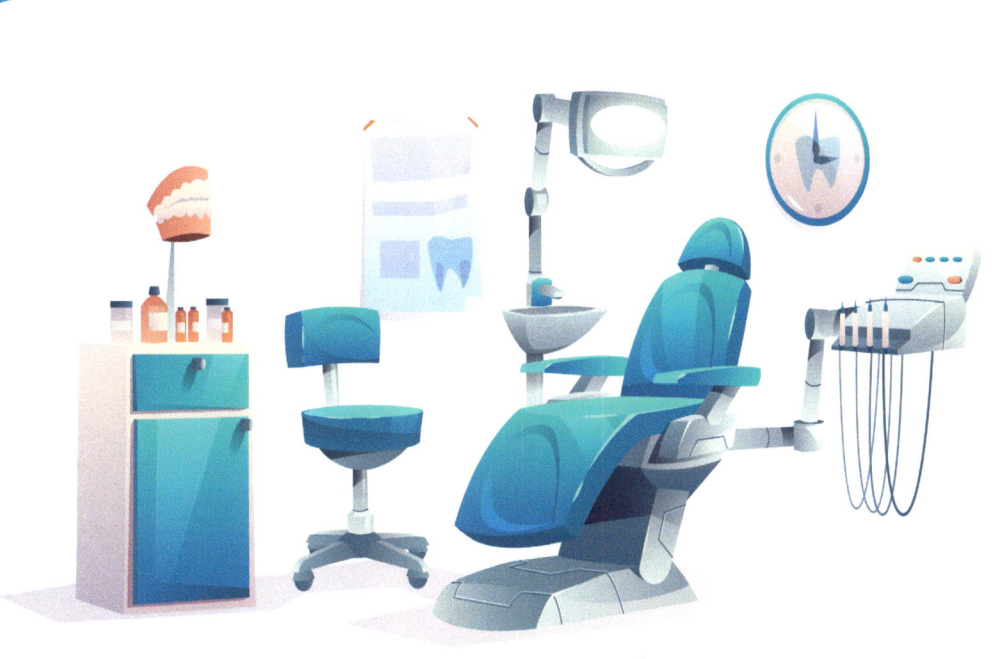

What kind of exciting things can you discover at the dental clinic?

The dental clinic is a special place where we go to take care of our teeth.

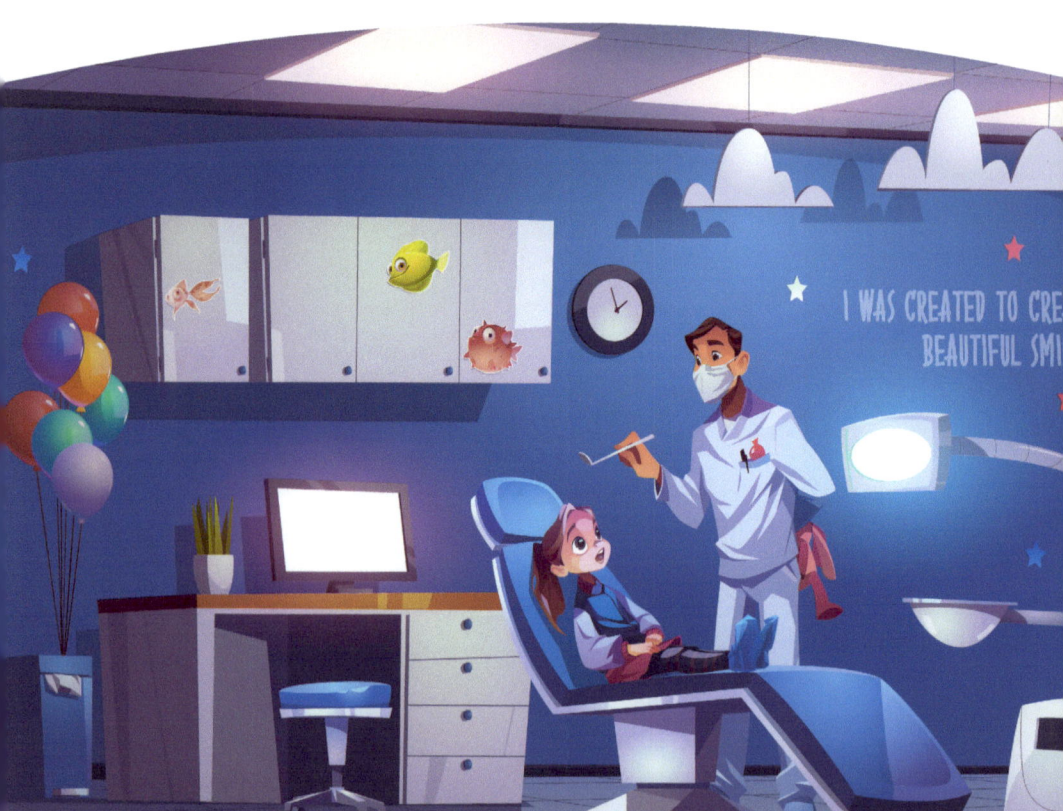

There are many interesting things to see and learn about at the dental clinic.

The dental Chair:

The dental chair is a special chair that moves up and down so that people of different sizes can sit in it comfortably.

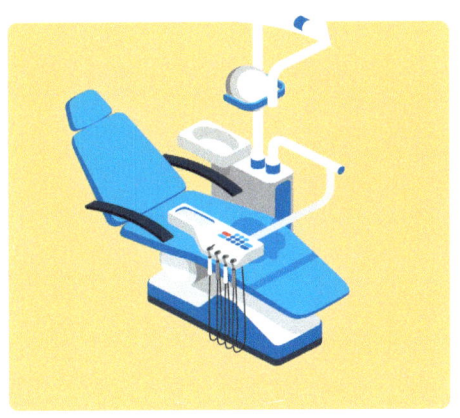

The dentist uses this chair to easily look into our mouths and check our teeth.

The dental lamp

The dental lamp is a special light that helps the dentist see inside our mouths clearly.

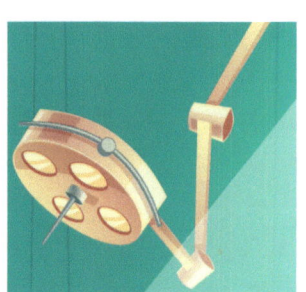

The dentist also uses special tools to take care of our teeth.

The dental mirror

The dental mirror is a small mirror that helps the dentist see our back teeth.

The "feeler"

The feeler helps the dentist count your teeth.

The tweezer

The tweezer is a tool that helps the dentist grab small things like cotton pieces.

The x-ray machine

The x-ray machine is a special machine that takes pictures of the inside of our teeth.

This helps the dentist see if we have any problems with our teeth that we can't see with our eyes.

The water spray and suction are tools that help the dentist clean our teeth and keep our mouths dry.

The suction

The suction removes the water from the mouth.

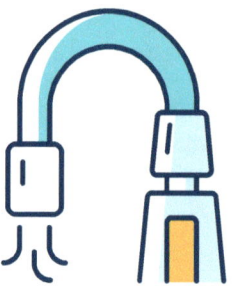

The water spray

The water spray sprays water into your mouth.

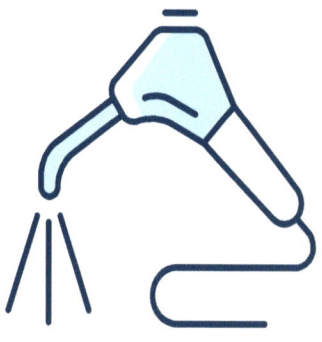

Let's Play

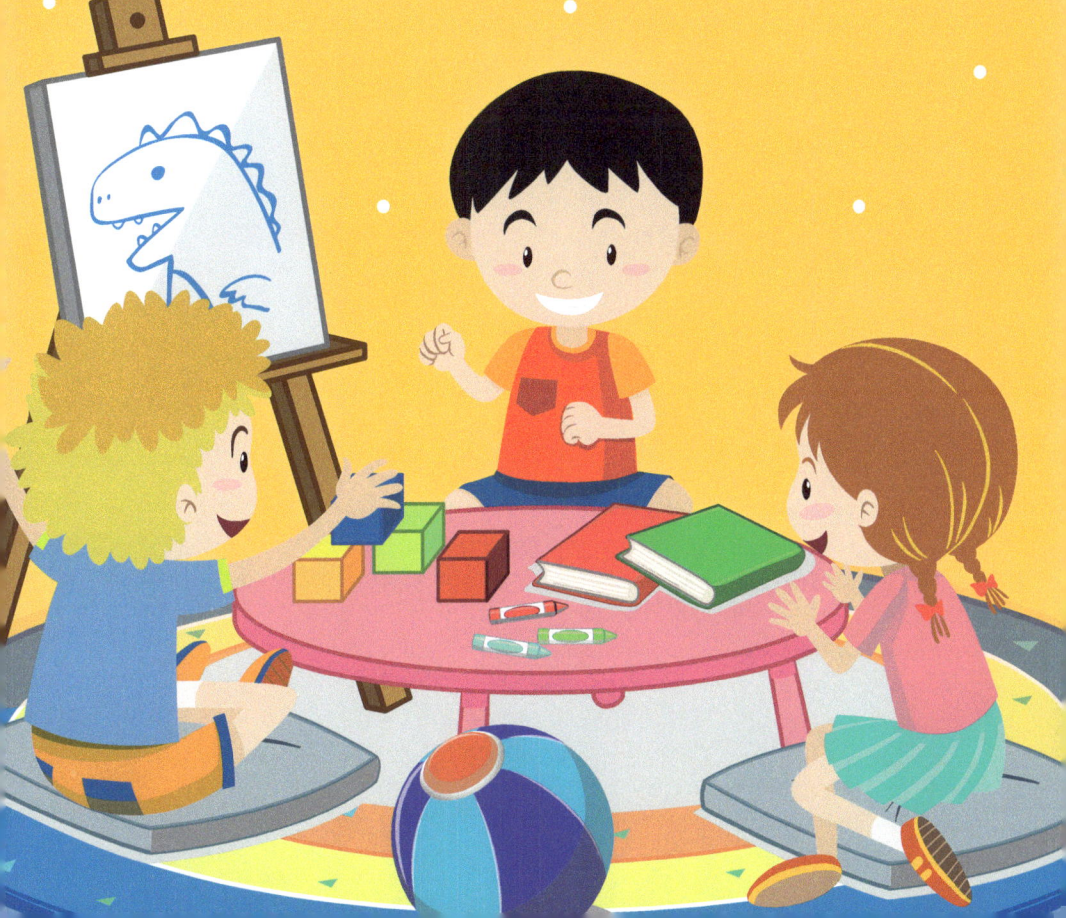

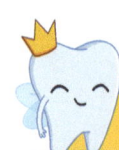 Color each picture the right color:

Yellow
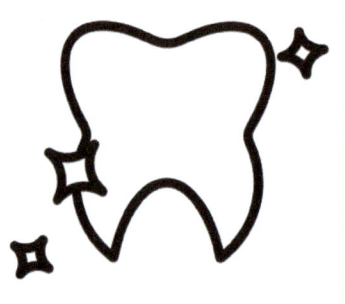

Blue
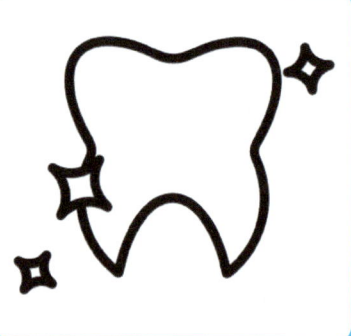

Green
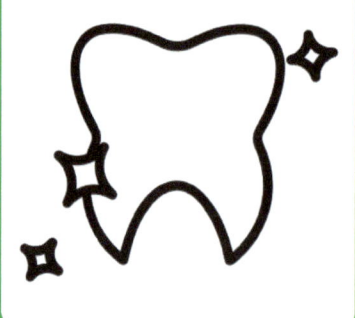

Red
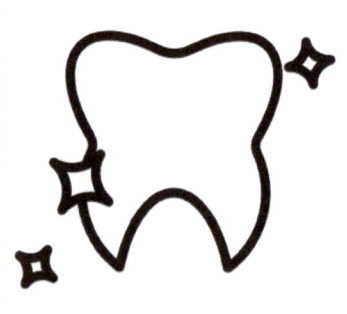

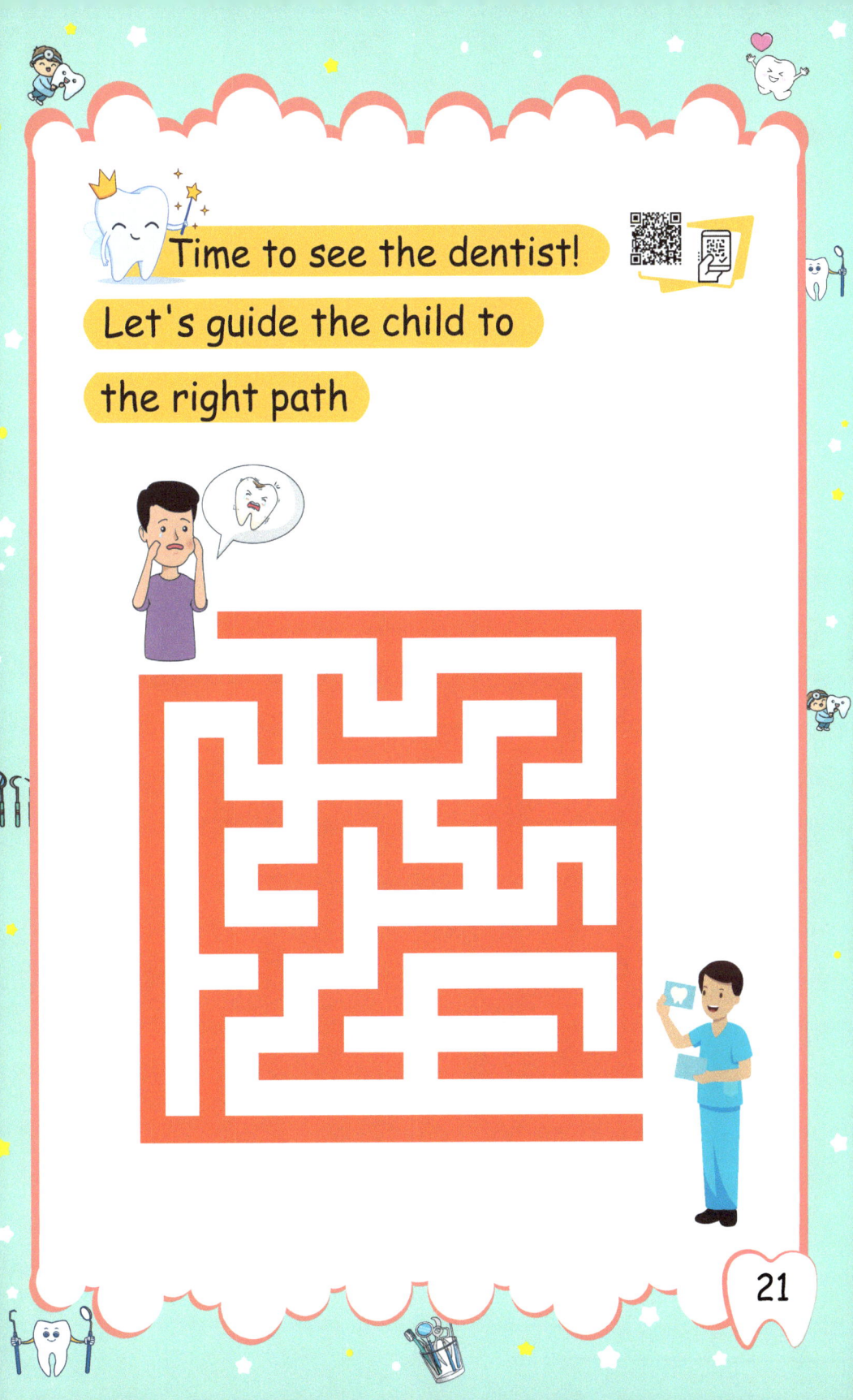

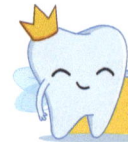 Match each picture with its label:

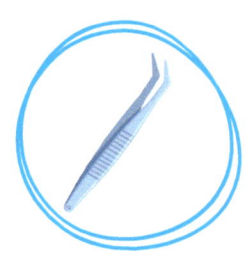 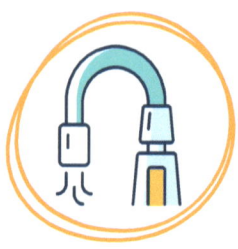 

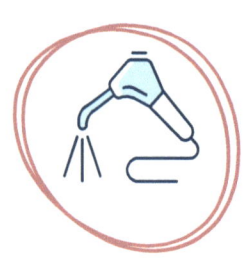 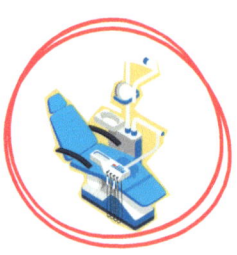 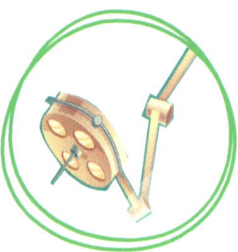

Dental Chair   Dental Mirror

Dental Lamp   Water Spray

Suction   Tweezer

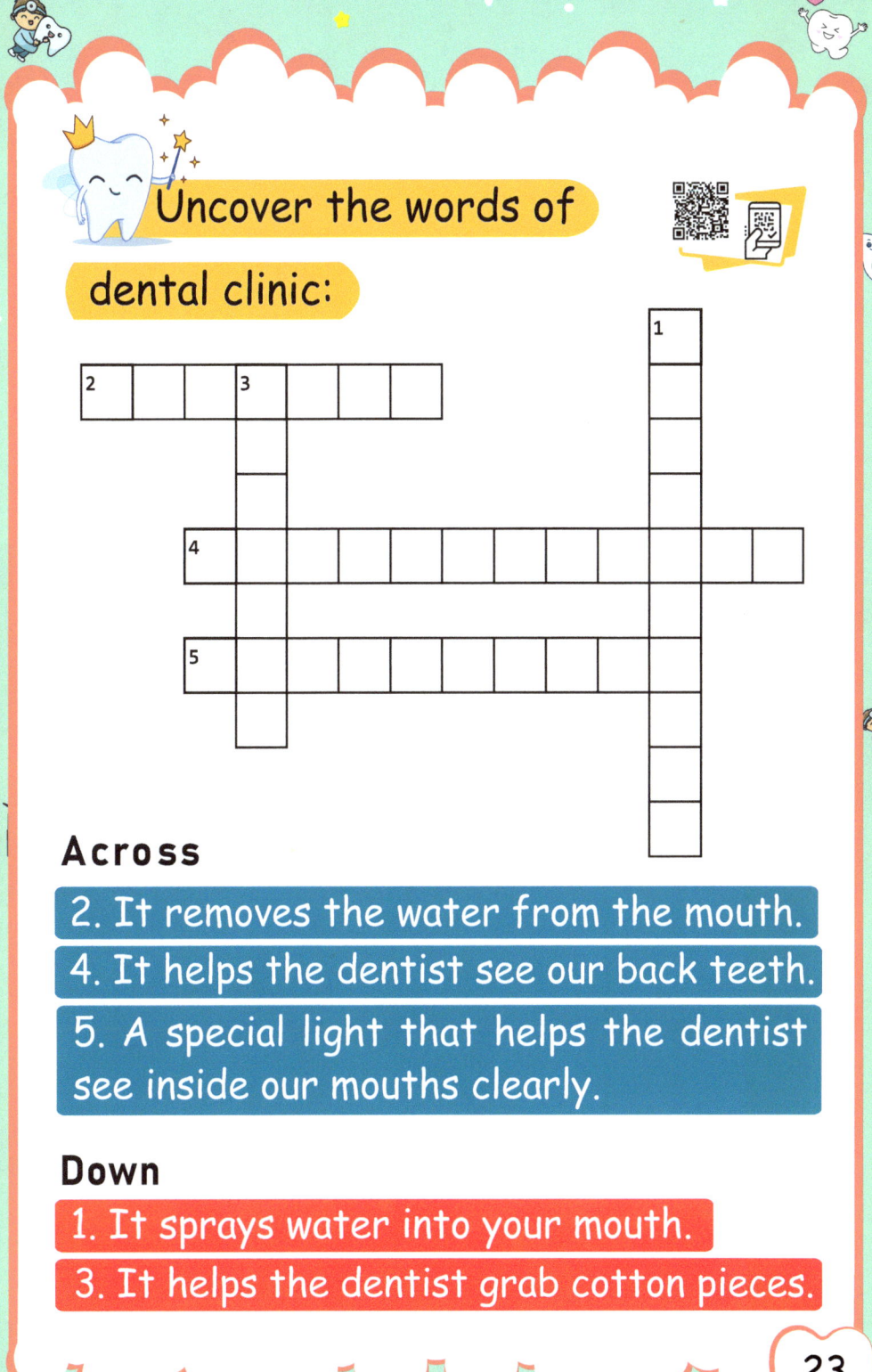

The Dental Team: The Friendly Faces Behind Your Smile

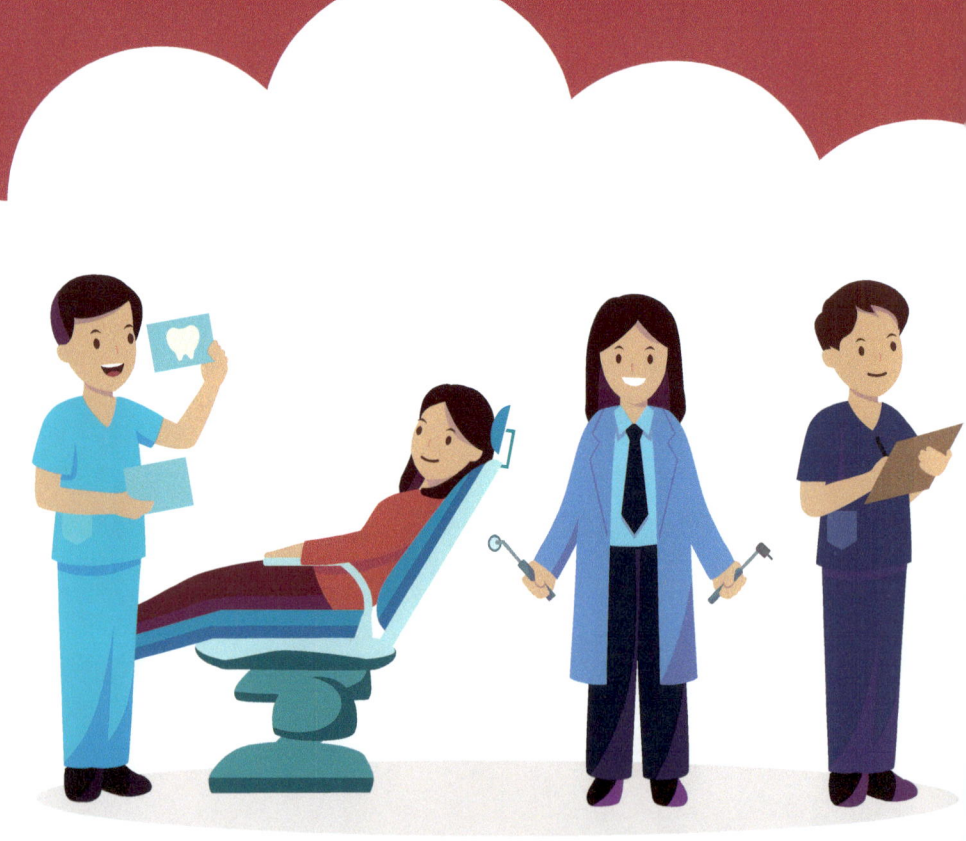

When you go to the dentist, you'll meet a team of helpers!

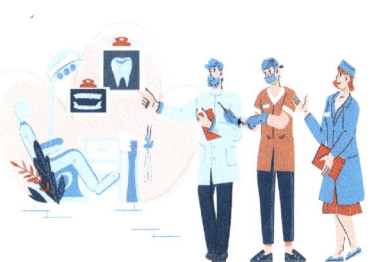

They all work together to make sure your teeth are healthy and strong.

Let's meet some of the members of the dental team!

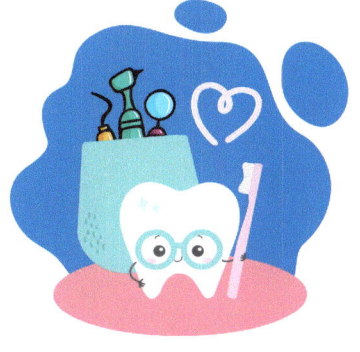

The receptionist

The receptionist is the first person you'll see when you come to the dental clinic.

They will greet you with a smile and help you check in for your appointment.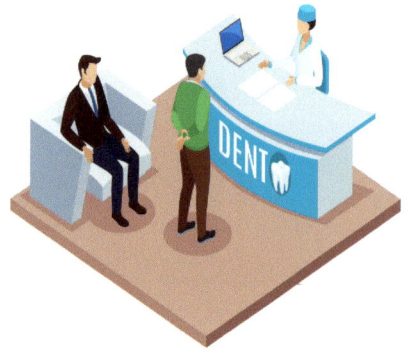

They might ask you some questions about your visit, and they might even give you a sticker or a toy to play with while you wait.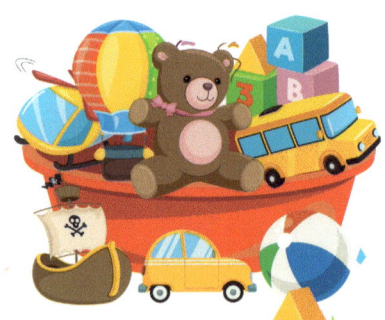

The dental assistant

The dental assistant is another important member of the dental team.

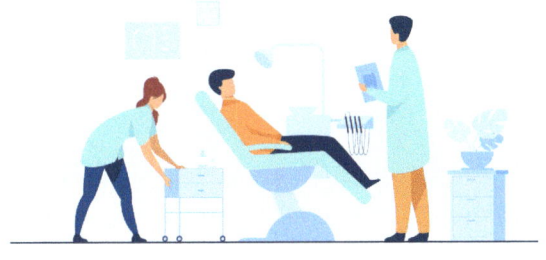

They help the dentist by getting the exam room ready for your visit.

They will make sure everything is clean and organized, and they might even help you get comfortable in the dental chair.

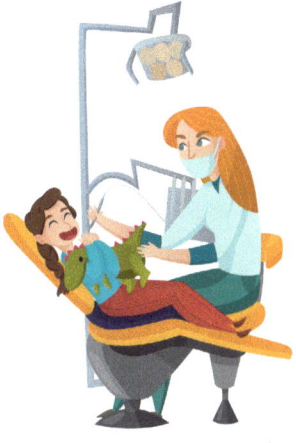

They might give you a special bib to wear, or they might put a blanket over your lap to keep you warm.

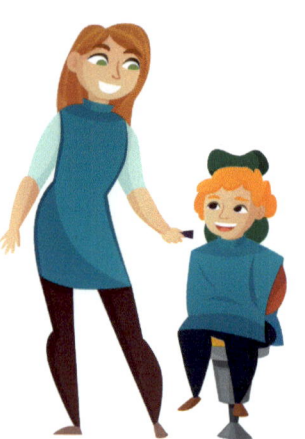

So the next time you visit the dental clinic, remember that the dental team is here to help you.

They are friendly, kind, and they want you to have healthy, shining teeth.

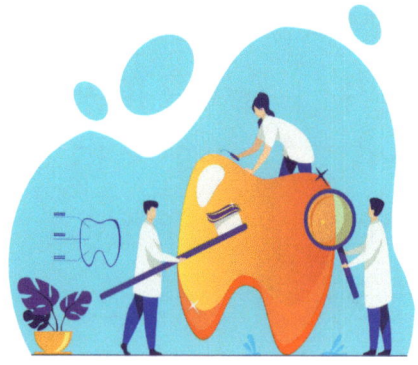

Let's Play

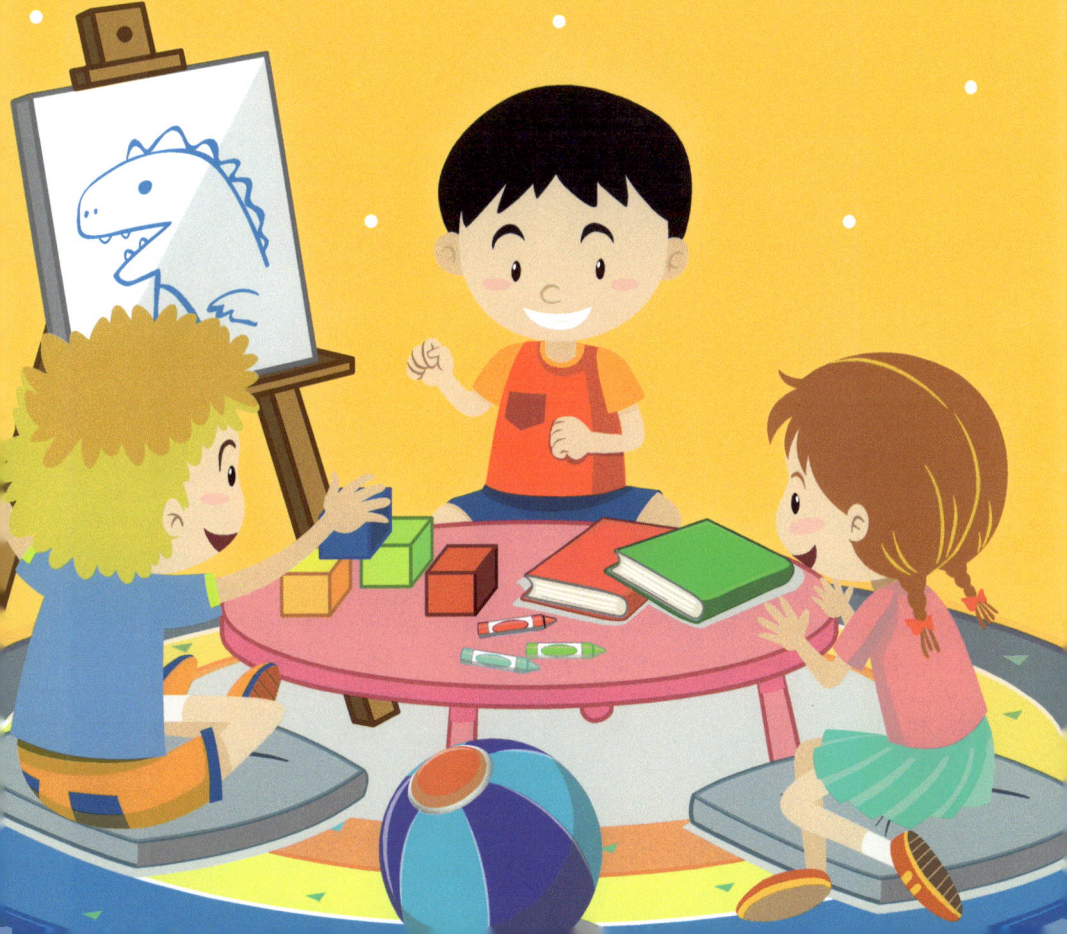

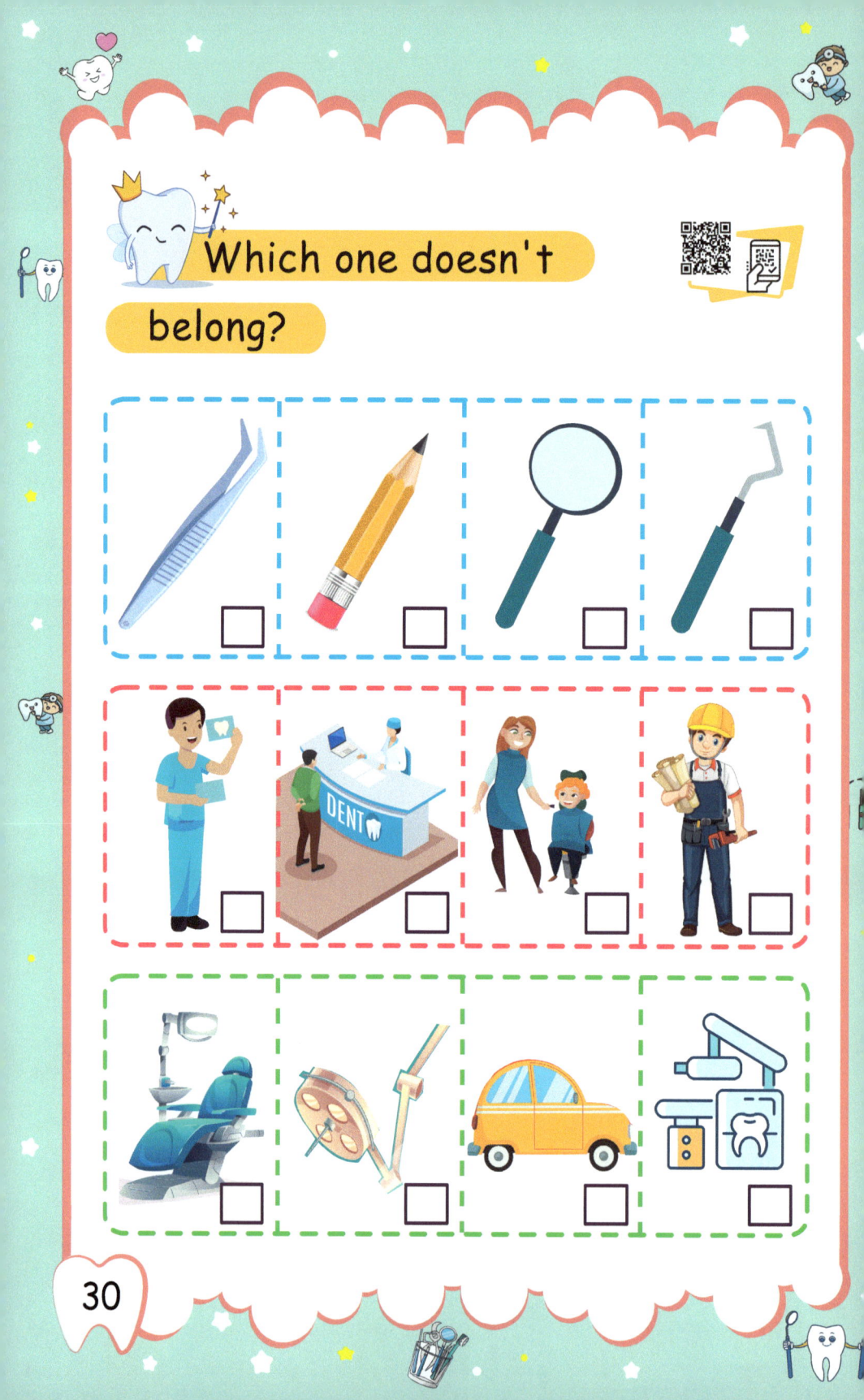

Match the Dental Team Members and Their Roles:

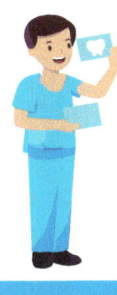

The Dentist

Fixes teeth problems

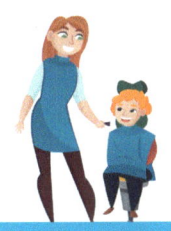

The Dental Assistant

Welcomes patients

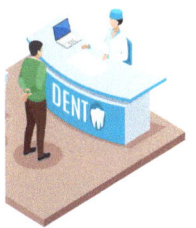

The Receptionist

Helps the dentist

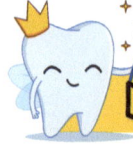

Dental Discovery

Word Search:

U	U	V	I	S	U	C	T	I	O	N	D
W	A	T	E	R	S	P	R	A	Y	A	Y
R	E	C	E	P	T	I	O	N	I	S	T
G	I	N	D	E	N	T	I	S	T	X	L
R	U	R	E	T	W	E	E	Z	E	R	Q
D	M	A	S	S	I	S	T	A	N	T	K
A	Z	O	C	Y	F	E	E	L	E	R	A
F	I	A	D	E	N	T	I	S	T	N	G

Find the following words in the puzzle:

- RECEPTIONIST
- WATER SPRAY
- ASSISTANT
- FEELER
- DENTIST
- TWEEZER
- SUCTION

32

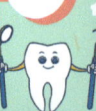

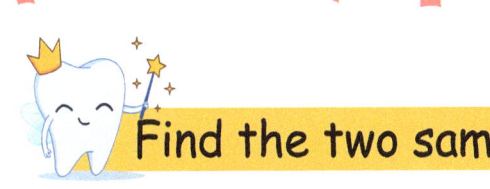 Find the two same toothbrushes.

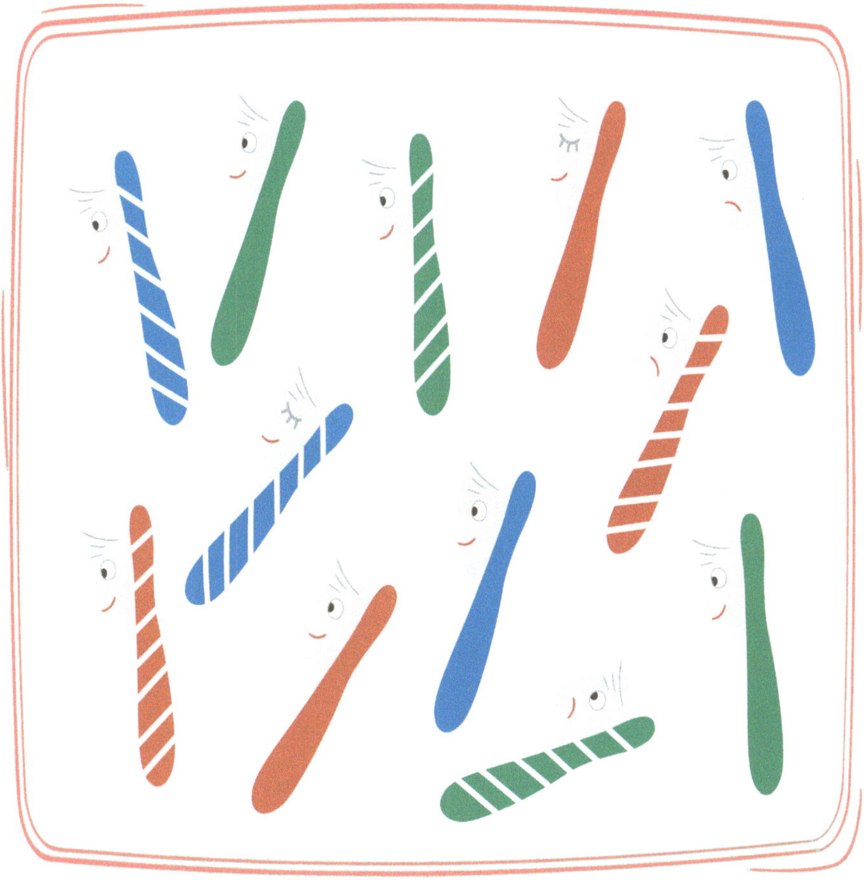

Guide to the parents

About the book:

This book is designed to guide your child through the process of a dental visit, including familiarizing them with the dental team and the tools they use. It also emphasizes the importance of regular check-ups and maintaining good oral hygiene for a healthy smile.

By the end of the book, your child will have a better understanding of:

• The importance of regular dental check-ups.
• The different roles of the dental team.
• The tools and equipment used by dentists during a check-up.

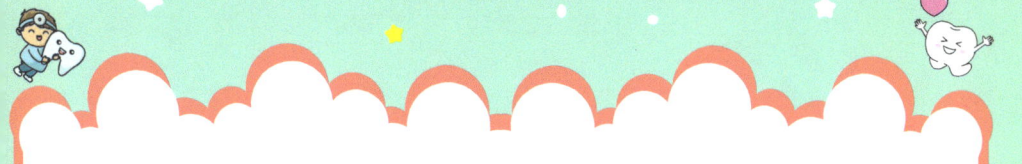

To get the most out of this interactive book, we recommend the following:

• Preview the book before reading it with your child to familiarize yourself with the content.

• Bring energy and enthusiasm to your reading sessions with your child.

• Take breaks to ask your child questions and discuss what you've read together.

• Use the games and activities provided at the end of each section to assess your child's comprehension.

• Consider revisiting the book with your child for added reinforcement.

• Take advantage of the QR codes provided throughout the book. These codes can be scanned with a smart device for an interactive and fun learning experience.

Some helpful dental information:

1. The first dental visit should take place around the age of one or when the first tooth erupts. This visit is important to establish a dental home and to begin preventative care.

2. Before the first visit, it's important to prepare your child for what to expect. You can read books about going to the dentist or watch videos together to help them understand the process.

3. During the visit, the dentist will examine your child's teeth and gums, check for proper eruption and spacing, and discuss proper oral hygiene techniques with you.

4. It's important to establish a regular schedule of dental check-ups, typically every six months, to maintain good oral

health and catch any issues early.

5. Remember, a positive attitude and open communication with your child's dentist can make all the difference in making dental visits a positive experience for both you and your child.

www.ingramcontent.com/pod-product-compliance
Lightning Source LLC
Chambersburg PA
CBHW040254220526
45473CB00001B/471